Understanding Garlic

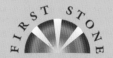

F I R S T   S T O N E

Contents

Foreword

Glorious garlic! One of Mother Nature's most useful gifts to both ancient and modern society – and how amazing that, even today, garlic is still revealing secrets that have been kept locked up in the magic clove for centuries!

Understanding Garlic gives an excellent summary of the wonderful characteristics of fresh and processed garlic, revealing its truly fascinating history, and how, in recent years, garlic has begun to live up to the reputation of a genuinely useful natural medicine.

Many an old wives' tale has been told about the powers of garlic, but this informative, interesting and valuable little book will amaze, entertain and reinforce the fact that garlic has an incredible cascade of benefits, and, when taken in the correct form, can really help to combat modern ailments.

Enjoy a clove or two today!

Peter Josling
The Garlic Information Centre

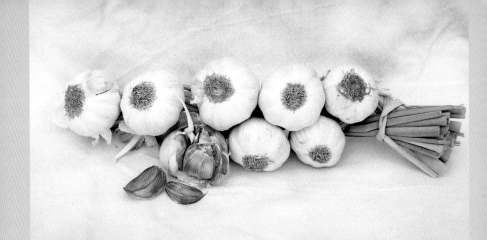

1

Introducing
Garlic

Gourmets and health gurus have revered garlic for thousands of years.

Unparalleled as a flavour enhancer and unequalled for its diverse healing benefits, garlic is one of nature's great masterpieces.

Indeed, when Hippocrates made his legendary statement "let food be your medicine, and medicine be your food" over 2,000 years ago, garlic was surely his inspiration.

For thousands of years, garlic has been used in the following ways:
- To flavour food.
- To cure fevers.

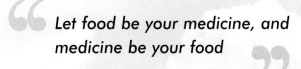

Let food be your medicine, and medicine be your food

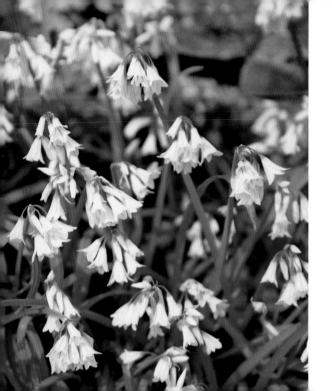

Garlic was first found growing in the deserts of Central Asia.

- To protect against vampires and witches.
- To bolster armies.
- To heal wounds.
- To treat infections and ailments, ranging from the plague, to heart disease and cancer.

THE HISTORY OF GARLIC

Although the exact location is unknown, garlic is believed to have originated in the deserts of Central Asia around Siberia.

The first historical evidence of garlic was found in cave dwellings over 10,000 years old. Sketches and clay sculptures of the bulb were found in Egyptian tombs dating back 5,700 years.

CHINESE MEDICINE

The first written evidence was found in an ancient Chinese text.

This relates the legend of the Yellow Emperor (over 4000BC) who ate a poisonous plant called yu-yu, but was saved by eating suan (garlic), which was found growing nearby.

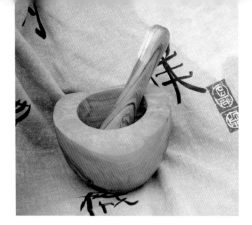

Garlic plays an integral part in Chinese Medicine.

The Yellow Emperor was one of the founding fathers of Traditional Chinese Medicine, and garlic has remained a very important remedy to this day in the ancient art of Chinese Medicine.

WESTERN WORLD
In the West, the first written evidence of garlic's special powers is traced back to Ancient Egypt. The Ebers Papyrus of 1500BC, recommended it as a

GARLIC TO THE RESCUE

In the Middle Ages, garlic was used to prevent the plague, and cloves were hung around the neck to ward off demons – and the occasional vampire.

treatment for 22 ailments.

The Pharaohs were quick to catch on to the benefits of garlic; they fed it to the slaves building their pyramids to increase their stamina and keep them in good general health.

The slaves obviously became converts, as ancient writings claim they went on strike when daily garlic rations were stopped.

The Israelites missed garlic when they were forced to flee Egypt and had to spend many years in the desert with Moses. "We remember the garlic which we did eat in Egypt…" (Numbers 11:5).

WARTIME
In more recent times, its use as an antiseptic saved tens of thousands of British soldiers' lives.

During the 1914-18 war, sterilised sphagnum moss soaked in garlic juice was used to treat suppurating wounds.

It was also used extensively on the Eastern Front during the Second World War, earning the nickname Russian Penicillin.

GARLIC – A VICTIM OF FASHION
Throughout the centuries, garlic has been in and out of fashion.

The ancient Romans thought garlic was strictly for consumption by the lower orders.

In Britain, Shakespeare called garlic the food of rustics.

The French have always had a high regard for garlic. Following a visit to France, the poet Shelley wrote of his surprise that young women of rank ate garlic.

THE STINKING ROSE

Many people shunned garlic because of its pungent odour, hence its nickname 'the stinking rose'.

King Henry IV of France used to chew raw cloves like sweets and reputedly had a breath that could 'fell an ox at 50 paces'. Nonetheless, he was reportedly still very popular with the ladies!

Wise people use the pungency of garlic to their advantage, as an old Yiddish saying testifies: "A dime will get you on the subway. Garlic will get you a seat."

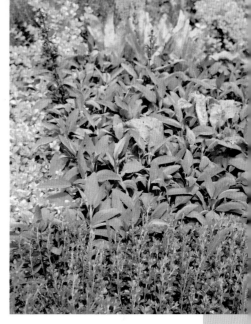

Herbs go in and out of fashion – but none more so than garlic.

13

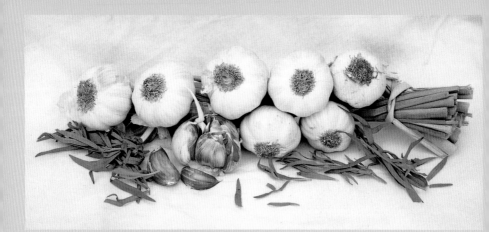

2

The Chemistry of Garlic

Garlic – allium sativum – is a member of the lily family. It had its first whiff of medical credibility in 1858 when Louis Pasteur discovered that its juice killed bacteria.

Since then, over 1,500 scientific studies have proved what folklore has known for thousands of years – garlic is highly successful at treating a wide variety of ailments.

Scientists have been striving to find out what makes garlic so successful as an 'adaptogen', a substance that brings the body back to its natural equilibrium. However, the more the chemical compounds in garlic are studied, the more complex they appear.

SULPHUR COMPOUNDS

These are the most studied of all of the compounds in garlic. They can generally be broken down into five groups.

❶ STABLE COMPOUNDS

Stable, odourless compounds, such as aliin, are found in unbroken garlic cloves. These are derivatives of the natural, sulphur-rich amino acid 'cysteine'.

❷ *INTERMEDIATES*

Intermediate compounds are formed whenever garlic is crushed, chopped or sliced. Their job is to release the enzyme aliinase, which, in turn, reacts with the odourless compounds (such as aliin) to make more complex sulphur compounds like 'allicin'.

Little is known about these intermediate 'shooting stars' because they disappear in a nano second and cannot be stored, even at low temperatures.

❸ *REACTIVE COMPOUNDS*

Allicin is a typical example of garlic's unstable, reactive compounds. These are formed by the combustion of the intermediates described above.

Allicin is one of nine 'chemical cousins' that give garlic its famous taste and odour, found in fresh garlic juice and in the air above chopped garlic.

While these compounds are

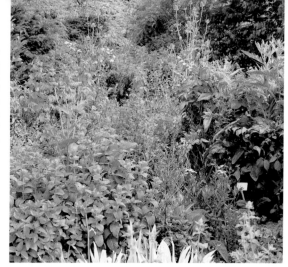

The healing power of herbs is well documented in folklore, but now scientific studies are underlining their value

unstable at room temperature, they can be prepared in pure form and can then be studied in the laboratory.

Allicin is regarded as the 'mother substance' of garlic, and is the most studied of all its compounds.

17

❹ OIL-BASED DERIVATIVES

When reactive compounds, such as allicin, are mixed with edible oils and allowed to stand at room temperature for more than a few hours, stable compounds of garlic are formed.

A good example of this situation is 'macerate of garlic'. Macerate is made when chopped garlic is mixed with edible oils.

This 'macerate of garlic' is known to be a rich source of naturally formed compounds, such as ajoene, methyl ajoene and dithiins.

❺ WATER-BASED DERIVATIVES

When garlic is heated in boiling water and the steam is condensed, distilled oil of garlic is produced. Diallyl disulphide is the scientific name for the major component of distilled oil of garlic. It has a strong 'chemical' smell of garlic, and is often used as a food flavouring agent.

NON-SULPHUR COMPOUNDS

Apart from its volatile oils, garlic contains vitamins A, C, E and B. It is a rich source of minerals, especially selenium, zinc and phosphorous. It also contains glucokinins, mucilage and germanium.

Germanium is present in garlic at the rate of 754 ppm (parts per million). Germanium stimulates the production of interferon, a powerful immune-enhancing chemical.

Interferon, in turn, improves the function of T-lymphocytes (free radical scavengers), B-lymphocytes (antibody manufacturers), and boosts the activity of natural killer cells.

Although a number of scientists strive to isolate individual healing compounds in garlic, many consider that it is the synergy of all of the compounds that account for its huge success as a 'pungent panacea'.

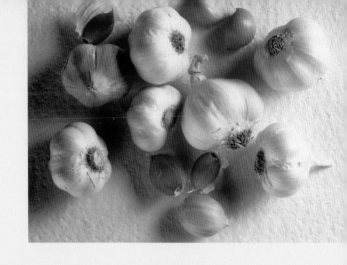

3

A Modern Day Wonder Drug

A yurvedic practitioners acknowledged garlic's abilities long ago when they named it 'mahanshadha', which in ancient Sanskrit means 'remedy for all diseases'.

In fact, the healing powers of garlic are so diverse that had it been made in the laboratory instead of by nature, it would probably be a high-priced prescription drug.

HEALING POWERS

The naturally occurring compounds in garlic make it a potent antioxidant, protecting cell membranes and DNA from damage and disease. In addition to acting as a protector, it also directly attacks bacteria and viruses while at the same time stimulating the body's natural defences against invaders.

In addition, garlic has the following powers:

- It reduces the clotting of blood platelets.
- It lowers blood cholesterol levels.
- It has an antiseptic, anti-

inflammatory and anti-fungal action.

- It has direct anti-tumour activity, inhibiting malignant cell growth.

Garlic has been successful in the treatment of intestinal putrefaction, fevers, parasites, high blood pressure, colic, fungal infections, dysentery, ulcers, worms, bacteria, viral infections, acne, tumours, diabetes, cholesterol… the list is endless.

Because of its success at treating so many ailments, garlic has become one of the most studied of all herbs. Case study findings show how successful garlic is at treating many different conditions.

GARLIC AND THE COMMON COLD

The Garlic Centre in East Sussex U.K. (further information, page 59) conducted an experiment with a total of 146 volunteers. Half of the volunteers took one capsule of an allicin supplement, while the remaining volunteers were given a placebo. Subjects were monitored over a 90-day period during the winter months. Only 24 colds were recorded amongst those taking the supplement, compared to 65 amongst those taking the placebo.

The study also found that among those who did catch a cold while taking the supplement, recovery time was speedier, and the chance of re-infection following a cold was significantly reduced.

Professor Eccles of the Common Cold Centre at Cardiff University thought this was 'a very encouraging study'.

GARLIC AND FUNGAL INFECTIONS

Many naturopathic practitioners routinely prescribe raw garlic and garlic supplements to patients with intestinal candidiasis. Another type of fungus that responds well to garlic therapy is athlete's foot.

In both cases, raw garlic can be used topically: in the case of intestinal candidiasis it is administered as a pessary, and with athlete's foot, slices of garlic are placed directly on the location of the infection, then bandaged to hold the slices in place.

GARLIC AND CANCER

Most studies have focused on the use of garlic as a cancer preventive, or its ability to influence pre-cancerous conditions. An example of one of these studies was carried out at the Nanjing Cancer Institute.

Certain parts of China have a much higher incidence of cancer of the stomach and oesophagus. The NCI compared the incidence of these cancers among thousands who ate lots of garlic, versus an equal number who ate little or none.

- There was a 70 per cent reduction in cancer of the oesophagus in those who ate lots of garlic.
- There was a 69 per cent reduction in cancer of the stomach in those who ate lots of garlic.
- There was no significant

reduction in the control group.

Garlic is believed to stimulate the production of the antioxidant 'glutathione', and the cancer-blocking enzyme cascade known as 'Cytochrome P-450'. One other explanation is that garlic stops the transformation of nitrates into highly carcinogenic nitrosamines.

In fact, there is a current research project to determine whether garlic offers any protection from the carcinogens in chargrilled hamburgers!

GARLIC AND CHOLESTEROL

A study in India followed two groups of males aged between 18-35 who had never eaten garlic before. (In India, there are sections of the population who traditionally do not eat garlic.)

One group was given 10 grams of raw garlic a day, while the other group ate as normal, i.e. no garlic. The study lasted two months.

Blood samples were taken at

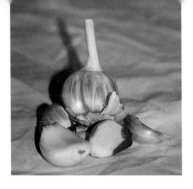

A case study proved that eating raw garlic lowers cholesterol levels.

the beginning and end of the study to monitor any changes in cholesterol levels.

Initially, cholesterol ranges were between 160-250 mg%. At the end of the two-month study, these ranges had decreased significantly in all subjects in the experimental (garlic) group, while the control group showed no significant decrease.

It was concluded that consuming 10 grams of raw garlic a day could successfully lower cholesterol, even when it was within normal range. Other studies have shown that garlic is not only able to reduce levels of the harmful

LDL (low density lipoprotein) cholesterol, but to increase levels of the beneficial HDL (high density lipoprotein).

GARLIC AND THE CARDIOVASCULAR SYSTEM

In a double blind placebo-controlled study to test garlic's ability to reduce arterial plaque, 152 individuals were followed for four years.

Group A was given 900mg of supplemental garlic daily, while group B was given no garlic at all. At the end of the four-year period, researchers reported a reduction in atherosclerotic deposits of up to 50 per cent in group A, while there was no significant reduction in any of the subjects in group B.

It was concluded that long-term use of garlic could successfully reduce atherosclerosis at a dosage of 900mg per day.

A further, similar study noted that a temporary rise in high blood pressure and cholesterol may be noted as the fatty deposits were removed from the bloodstream.

Researchers concluded that

cardiovascular improvements through garlic supplementation would not happen overnight.

Other studies have shown that garlic discourages blood platelets from becoming sticky (so long as they are 'slippery', platelets won't clot), and that garlic also inhibits clot formation by increasing fibrinolytic activity (the breakdown of a clot before it becomes big enough to cause problems).

Many researchers believe that garlic blocks blood clot formation more effectively than aspirin. It also scores against aspirin in its ability to break down existing clots. Aspirin does not have this ability.

GARLIC AND BACTERIA

Studies conducted on the allicin compound in garlic show that it can kill 23 types of bacteria, including salmonella, campylobacter, helicobacter and staphylo-coccus. It is thought that its power to block the enzymes responsible for the metabolism of micro-organisms is responsible for this ability.

Professor Al Lastovica of

UCT explains that "these findings are of more than passing interest because many bacteria are becoming increasingly resistant to the antibiotics commonly used in treating bacterial infections".

Of great interest is the fact that garlic has proved effective at treating infections caused by the hospital superbug MRSA.

GARLIC AND PREGNANCY

Research has concluded that taking garlic during pregnancy can reduce the risk of pre-eclampsia (high blood pressure and protein retained in the urine). The same research team has also shown that garlic can help to increase the birth weight of babies destined to be too small. The obstetrics and gynaecology unit at Westminster and Chelsea hospital in London carried out this research.

It concluded that although pre-eclampsia and growth retardation are complex and multifactorial conditions, taking standardised garlic capsules throughout pregnancy may decrease the risk of these types of birth complications.

Furthermore, the activity of

key enzymes that are often low in abnormal pregnancies were significantly increased when garlic was supplemented.

NB: Because of the increased risk of internal bleeding, garlic should be taken with caution during pregnancy.

GARLIC AND IMPOTENCE

Garlic has always been known as an aphrodisiac, and, from a medical point of view, we know it can improve blood circulation significantly. Now it appears that an enzyme called nitric oxide synthase (NOS) is primarily responsible for the mechanism of erection.

Recent studies have shown that certain preparations of garlic can stimulate the production of NOS, particularly in individuals who have low levels of this enzyme. Science is again proving what folklore has always known!

OTHER STUDIES

In a Russian study, garlic was used as an inhalent to successfully treat over 200 cases of lung tuberculosis. Dr William Minchin lists other successful case studies on tuberculosis in his book *The Treatment of Tuberculosis with Oleum Allium*.

Another interesting case study comes from Australia, where garlic was found to cure ringworm infections three times faster than modern drugs.

Garlic has also been shown to be effective as an insect repellent – studies have proved its effectiveness against ticks, mosquitoes and fleas. Organic farmers often use garlic spray as an insecticide.

NEGATIVE RESEARCH

I tend to be slightly sceptical if I read completely negative research on garlic. Two questions immediately spring to mind:

- Does the research sponsor have a vested interest in the outcome?

- Have they used a high-quality supplement?

If you read an article claiming "Garlic Has No Health Benefits", ask yourself the same questions.

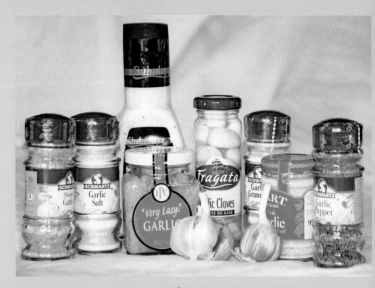

4 Using Garlic

The debate over the comparable benefits of raw or cooked garlic has raged for many years.

It was generally considered that cooked garlic lost most of its healing powers. It has since been discovered that the significance lies not in the cooking, but in the preparation.

If garlic is either cut, chopped, sliced, or crushed – and allowed to stand for at least ten minutes before being heated – not only will it retain its healing properties, it will gain more.

Once heated, the allicin in garlic prepared in this way will produce substances called ajoene and DADS (diallyl disulphide) that can prevent blood from clotting.

GETTING THE MOST FROM YOUR GARLIC

- Buy organic: if you want garlic to boost your health, it doesn't make any sense to buy cloves that have been grown on a bed of chemical fertiliser and sprayed with toxic pesticides.

- Make sure the garlic is as

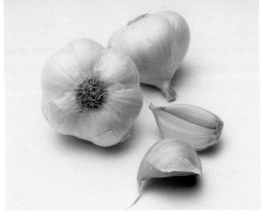

Don't peel garlic until you are ready to use it.

fresh as possible. Fresh cloves are solid and firm to the touch.

• Store it in a cool dry place, in a container that allows the air to circulate.

• Do not peel the cloves until you need to use them. Peeled cloves become mouldy quicker.

• If you make (or buy) oil-based dressing using garlic,

be sure to keep it in the fridge and do not store for more than two weeks. Garlic is very alkaline, and when stored in oil, it is very susceptible to botulism.

IS ALL GARLIC THE SAME?

There are more than 300 different strains of garlic grown all over the world. They vary in colour from white to dark wine shades. Some bulbs have fat cloves, while others have skinny cloves.

Although garlic is a root crop, there are strains where the bulbs grow above the ground. 'Elephant garlic' is not really garlic: it's a leek.

The top producer of garlic is China, which accounts for 66 per cent of the world's garlic every year. The Shandong Province, which is a prime agricultural area, south-east of Beijing, leads the field. South Korea and India are second and third respectively with 5 per cent each. The USA ranks fourth, with 3 per cent of the world's production.

The strength of garlic is

rated on its 'allicin potential'. Allicin is regarded as being the active ingredient in garlic, but as no allicin is produced until the cloves are broken, only the 'potential' for allicin can be measured. This is achieved by measuring the stable sulphur compounds that will convert into allicin. Allicin potential can vary as much as 13 fold.

Chinese garlic has the highest allicin potential at 6 per cent, while Egyptian garlic has much less than 0.03 per cent. As Egypt is one of the largest exporters in the world, it is worth finding out where your garlic comes from. Interestingly, if Chinese garlic is grown outside China, its allicin potential falls. Many garlic supplements also use 'allicin potential' as a guide to potency.

CLOVES OR PILLS?

Will a clove a day keep disease at bay? Many researchers feel that a clove a day is okay as prevention, but generally not enough if you want to reverse a pre-existing condition. A therapeutic dose of garlic

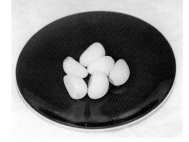

Eating raw garlic is not a realistic option for most people.

could be ten cloves a day.

Now, unless you live alone, don't socialise, and have the digestive system of an ox, it's pretty difficult to consume that amount of fresh garlic daily. People want the benefits of garlic without the side-effects, which include: heartburn, flatulence, increased pulse, and smelly breath.

They are also prepared to pay for it: the world market for garlic supplements is now approaching £200million per annum.

There is a staggering array of garlic supplements on sale, but they basically fall into five categories:

GARLIC OILS
This type of processing was developed about 70 years ago and was the first type of garlic supplement available.

Supplements contain minute amounts of essential oil, which has been steam distilled from raw garlic.

Although they contain none of the important water soluble compounds, have a strong garlic odour, and there is very little research to back up their claims, many people swear by the effectiveness of garlic oil supplements.

GARLIC OIL MACERATES
These supplements consist of raw garlic ground and mixed with vegetable oil. This

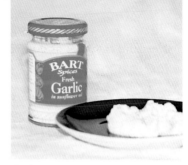

Garlic can be ground and mixed with vegetable oil.

produces substances called ajoene and dithiins, which are considered beneficial if you are at risk of strokes or thrombosis.

GARLIC POWDERS
Some of the market leaders

fall into this category, as do many supermarket 'own brand' and 'mail order' supplements. In addition to a small amount of oil-soluble compounds, garlic powders contain aliin and the enzyme allinase. The tablets are encased in an enteric coating, which stops the active enzyme from being destroyed by stomach acids.

Theoretically, this process allows allicin to be produced safely in the small intestine and reduces the infamous 'garlic breath'. However, not all manufacturers are equally rigorous in their production methods. A standardised high 'allicin yield' powder is considered optimal. Problems often associated with low yield and generally cheaper products are:

- They contain less 'allicin potential'.
- They generally contain more fillers and binders that inhibit enzyme activity.
- The enteric coatings often fail to break down properly.

There has been much positive

research on the ability of standardised high allicin yield powders to reduce cholesterol and high blood pressure.

AGED GARLIC EXTRACT

The manufacturers of AGE believe that ageing garlic in vinegar for up to 20 months increases the herb's potency. In fact, the Chinese have been doing this for centuries.

AGE doesn't contain allicin, but the well-researched S-allyl-cysteine and S-allyl-mercaptocysteine. It has the benefit of being odourless, and is available as a syrup. AGE supplements command more than half the world market in garlic supplements.

STABILISED ALLICIN

An Israeli company claims to have developed a method to stabilise allicin for supplementation. It is early days, but watch this space…

HOW MUCH GARLIC SHOULD I TAKE?

Based on clinical trials, a daily dose of a garlic supplement should provide at least 10mg alliin, or a total allicin 'potential' or 'yield' of

4,000mcg. This dosage equates to 4 grams, or one medium-sized clove of raw garlic a day.

It is not possible to rate the amount of 'aged garlic' with raw garlic as it contains compounds not found in raw garlic, but it is generally safe to follow the recommended daily dose. Therapeutic dosages can be much higher, but it is always best to take the advice of a health care practitioner as individual needs vary.

IS GARLIC SAFE?

Gastrointestinal irritation and nausea are the most frequent side-effects – apart from odour on the breath and skin for which the herb is so famous.

Because garlic can thin the blood, it is advisable to discuss taking supplements with your doctor if you are taking warfarin or any other anti-coagulant medication.

Garlic has also been shown to reduce the potential of certain HIV medications by up to 50 per cent. Obviously, this must be checked out with your doctor.

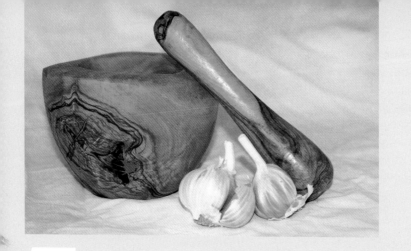

5 Common Ailments

Some years ago, Dr Christopher, the renowned naturopath, was called to the house of a dying toddler. The child had pneumonia and had been pronounced incurable by the family physician.

The distraught parents called everyone they knew to ask for help and someone suggested Dr Christopher.

When he arrived, Dr Christopher examined the child and proceeded with the following treatment:

- He massaged oil into the child's feet and up around the ankles.
- He then made up a paste of chopped garlic and vaseline (50:50).
- He applied the paste, about half an inch thick, to the soles of the child's feet.
- The feet were then loosely bandaged and covered with socks.

This was the only treatment Dr Christopher used.

The next morning, the family physician arrived,

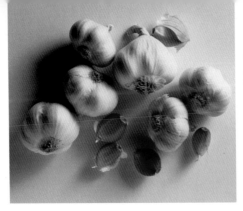

Garlic can have a remarkable effect on certain heart conditions.

thinking he would be signing the child's death certificate. He was shocked to see the child sitting in his highchair, eating his first food for days.

The physician was indignant that someone else had taken over and 'gone against procedure'. However, he left rather sheepishly when the parents asked if the outcome of 'proper procedure' would have resulted in the death of their son.

HELPLINE

While there is an abundance of anecdotal evidence on the use of garlic for bronchial conditions, you must refer someone to a doctor if you suspect a severe bronchial infection. Further information regarding Dr Christopher's remedies can be found in the resources section at the back of this book.

TRIED-AND-TESTED REMEDIES

A number of remedies have been tried and tested over a long period, and have proved to be of immense value.

In all cases, consult your doctor if the condition does not improve, or if you have any other concerns.

SORE THROAT AND COUGHS

- Mash all the cloves from a garlic bulb into a paste.
- Add six teaspoons of apple cider vinegar.

- Marinate overnight in a refrigerator.
- Next day, take a large tablespoon of honey (warm it gently if necessary), the juice of one lemon, and add it to the marinated mixture.
- Take two teaspoons of this mixture every morning.
- Keep it in the mouth until it becomes liquid, then allow it to trickle down the throat.
- Store the mixture in the fridge for one week, then discard.

WASP STINGS
- Rub a cut clove of garlic on to the area that has been stung. Within a few minutes, the pain and swelling will begin to disappear.

TOOTHACHE
- Cut a clove and place the cut end directly on the tooth.
- Hold it there until the pain eases, or disappears completely.

ENCOURAGING BREASTFEEDING
Babies stay longer at the breast when the mother eats garlic. They will also benefit

from the many healing properties of garlic in the breast milk.

ATHLETE'S FOOT, WARTS, VERRUCAS

- Place thick slices of garlic directly on the affected area/s, and keep in place with either gauze or a bandage.
- Repeat as necessary until the condition has disappeared.

EARACHE

- Prick a largish garlic clove and steep it in almond or olive oil for a few minutes.
- Place it gently in the hollow of the ear. Be careful not to penetrate the ear.

MOUTH ULCERS

- Chop the end off a clove of garlic.
- Dip it in natural yoghurt and hold against the ulcer. It will sting, but only momentarily.

NASAL CONGESTION

- Take four or five cloves, crush them, and add a little apple cider vinegar.
- Pour on a pint of boiling water and inhale the fumes.

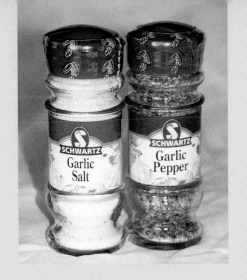

6 Recipes For Garlic Lovers

People generally have quite fixed ideas about garlic in food – they either love it or they hate it. Here are a couple of recipes for those who love it...

GARLIC CHICKEN

Ingredients
1 chicken, washed and cut into quarters
6 cloves of garlic
1½ tablespoons olive oil
Juice of 1 lemon
Sprinkle of oregano
Salt and pepper to taste.

Method
- Preheat the oven to 350 degrees F.
- Lightly oil a roasting dish.
- Cut half of the garlic into slithers.
- Pierce the skin of the chicken all over and slide the garlic slithers under the skin.
- Mash the rest of the garlic with the remaining oil and lemon juice.
- Rub this mixture over the chicken.
- Sprinkle with oregano, salt and pepper.

49

PERFECT GARLIC ROAST POTATOES

Ingredients
1 lb (0.4kg) of small white or red potatoes (peeled or not – your choice)
6 or 7 cloves of garlic
¼ cup olive oil
Salt and pepper to taste.

Method
- Preheat the oven to 350 degrees F.
- Wash potatoes, and peel if desired.
- Add salt to taste and boil for 10 minutes.
- Drain, put the lid on the pan, and shake to break the edges of the potatoes slightly. Allow to cool a little.
- While they are cooling, mash the garlic and mix to a paste with the oil, and add a little extra salt and pepper to taste, if desired.
- Once the potatoes have cooled sufficiently, rub the mixture around the potatoes.
- Put them in a roasting dish and bake on the top shelf of

the oven. Turn once or
twice during cooking.

- They will be ready in
  approximately 45 minutes.

LEMON-GARLIC SORBET

Ingredients

1 cup sugar
1 head of roasted, peeled
  garlic
Skin of 1 small lemon
Dash salt
3 cups water
⅔ cup lemon juice

To make about a quart.

Method

- In a food processor,
  combine sugar, roasted
  garlic, lemon skin, and salt.
  Process until the skin is
  finely chopped.
- Transfer to saucepan and
  add water.
- Heat just until the sugar
  dissolves.
- Cool, then add lemon juice.
- Cover and chill.
- Process in an ice-cream
  maker according to the
  manufacturer's directions.
- Store, tightly covered, in
  freezer.

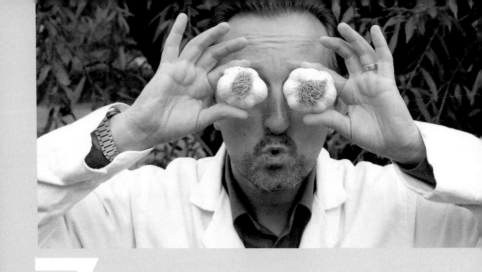

7 Fun Facts About Garlic

Rub some crushed garlic on the soles of someone's feet. Within five minutes you will be able to detect garlic odour on their breath.

Proof positive that garlic applied to the soles of the feet, as in Dr Christopher's remedy (see page 43), can reach the lungs. Be careful to apply oil first, as raw garlic can blister the skin.

FIGHTING FAT
Taking garlic supplements with a fatty meal can prevent absorption of the fat.

SLIM ON CALORIES
One clove of garlic contains between one and four calories.

CRACKING EGGS
Chickens lay bigger eggs if garlic is added to their feed.

DOCTOR'S ORDERS
Garlic is a prescription medicine in Germany, Holland and Denmark.

HORSE POWER
In France, horses are fed a diet of garlic and onions to reduce blood clots in the legs.

TOP CROP
Pink garlic, 'ail rose' from Lautrec in south-west France, has an 'appellation' guaranteeing its provenance and quality.

GROWING GOOD
One of the easiest varieties of garlic to grow comes from Clermont-Ferrand in France.

NEW CHANNEL
People in the south of England eat twice as much garlic as those in northern France.

NATURAL HIGH
In Tibet, the caravan men chew garlic as an antidote to altitude sickness.

SOUPER CURE
Chicken soup with garlic is known as 'Jewish penicillin'.

CROWS STONED
If crows eat garlic, it stupefies them.

CANCER FIGHTER
The director of the National Cancer Institute of America has said that garlic has more

potential than any other food as a cancer-fighting substance.

VAPOURISING GERMS

A report in *Science Weekly* magazine in Germany showed that freshly cut garlic could kill bacteria at a distance of 20 cm by its vapour alone.

IT'S IN THE BLOOD

A study in the late 90s showed that garlic might *attract* vampires!

As no vampire volunteers could be found, leeches were used instead.

When given the choice of a hand smeared with garlic or a clean hand, the leeches repeatedly chose the garlic hand in preference to the clean hand.

RED HOT NEWS

During a flu epidemic in Russia in 1965, the *Moscow Evening News* told everyone to "Eat more garlic!"

THE REAL VAMPIRES

The vampire legend is thought to have its origins in the

Middle Ages.

People with a condition known as 'porphyria' avoided garlic at all costs as it worsened their condition.

They had thin blood and were also photo (light) sensitive – the vampire connection is clear!

BEAUTIFUL GARLIC

The Koreans have a 'Miss Garlic' beauty contest every year.

FOOD FOR THOUGHT

The *American Journal of Clinical Nutrition* reported that when garlic bread is served at dinner, people argue less.

FOUR THIEVES

In France during the plague years, it was common for condemned prisoners to be forced to bury plague victims.

Usually their fate was sealed, but four such prisoners never succumbed to the plague.

It was discovered that they consumed large quantities of garlic soaked in wine vinegar.

To this day, the concoction is known as 'vinaigre des quatres voleurs' – four thieves vinegar.

A GREATER LOVE
In Latvia, it is illegal for a man to expect his wife to make love to him after eating garlic.

GATHERING'S GARLIC
In Berkeley, California, there is an organisation whose members gather monthly to honour the garlic plant. They are "The Lovers of the Stinking Rose".

YOU MUST REMEMBER THIS
Elinor Roosevelt ate three chocolate-flavoured garlic balls every day of her life because her doctor told her it would improve her memory.

JUST THE TICKET
In Indiana it is illegal to ride public transport for 30 minutes after eating garlic.

STUNNING STRING
The longest string of garlic stretched to 123 ft (35 metres). It was put together in 1996 in the English village of Catsfield in East Sussex.

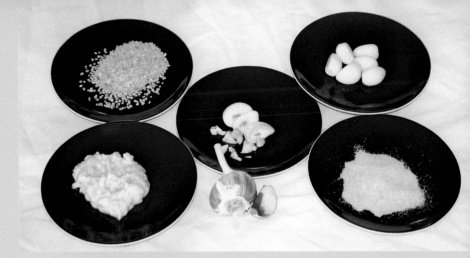

8 Further Information

Growing garlic, cooking with garlic, or using garlic as a remedy – there's lots more to know about this versatile herb.

THE GARLIC INFORMATION CENTRE

Tel: 01424 892440
Fax: 01424 892988
www.mistral.co.uk/garlic/

An international information service about the medicinal benefits of garlic.

BOOKS TO READ

• Herbal Home Health Care.
Author: Dr. John R. Christopher.
Publisher: Atlantic Books, 1976.

• All About Garlic.
Author: Stephen Fullder.
Publisher: Avery Publishing, 1999.

• The Garlic Lover's Cookbook.
Author: Gilroy Garlic Festival.
Publisher: Celestial Arts, 1980.

• Garlic, Garlic, Garlic: Exceptional recipes from the world's most indispensable ingredient.
Authors: Linda and Fred Griffith.
Publisher: Houghton Mifflin, 1998.

• Growing Great Garlic: The definitive guide for organic gardeners.
Author: Ron L. Engeland.
Publisher: Chelsea Green Publishing Company.

• Garlic: The Healing Herb: All about its remarkable range of medicinal and culinary properties.
Author: Paul Simons.
Publisher: Harper Collins, 1986.

• Garlic Lovers' Greatest Hits: 20 years of prize-winning recipes from the Gilroy Garlic Festival.
Author: Gilroy Garlic Festival.
Publisher: Celestial Arts, 1998.

The Totally Garlic Cookbook.
Authors: Helen Siegel and Karen Gillingham.
Publisher: Celestial Arts, 1994.

• The Great Garlic Book: A guide with recipes.
Author: Chester Aaron.
Publisher: Ten Speed Press, 1997.

• Garlic: The Natural Remedy.
Author: Karen Evennett.
Publisher: Ulysses Press, 1998.

• Garlic: How Garlic Protects Your Heart.
Author: Edzard Ernst.
Publisher: Amberwood, 1996.

• Garlic: Immunity Booster and Heart Helper.
Author: Stephanie Pedersen.
Publisher: Dorling Kindersley Publishing, 2000.

• The Healing Benefits of Garlic.
Author: John Heinerman.
Publisher: Random House, USA, Inc.

WEBSITES

• The Garlic Store
www.thegarlicstore.com
Online store providing information.

• The Garlic Shoppe
www.garlicshoppe.com
Online store.

• Garlic Lovers
www.garliclovers.com
Online store providing information and garlic-related products.

• Gourmet Garlic
www.gourmetgarlicgardens.com/health.htm
Information about the various health benefits of garlic.

• Garlic Health Benefits
www.garleo.com/article.htm
Information about health benefits.

About the author

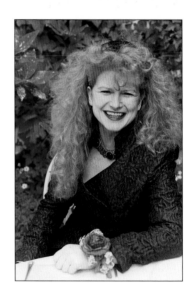

Marjorie Green is a practitioner,
writer and lecturer on Clinical
Nutrition, Bioenergetic Medicine,
Neuro Linguistic Programming and
Emotional Freedom Techniques. She
has made many appearances on
television and radio.

She can be contacted via e-mail:
marjoriecgreen@aol.com

Other titles in the series

- Understanding Acupressure
- Understanding Acupuncture
- Understanding The Alexander Technique
- Understanding Aromatherapy
- Understanding Bach Flower Remedies
- Understanding Echinacea
- Understanding Evening Primrose
- Understanding Feng Shui
- Understanding Fish Oils
- Understanding Ginseng
- Understanding Head Massage
- Understanding Kinesiology
- Understanding Lavender
- Understanding Massage
- Understanding Pilates
- Understanding Reflexology
- Understanding Reiki
- Understanding St. John's Wort
- Understanding Shiatsu
- Understanding Yoga

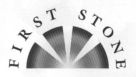

First published 2003 by First Stone Publishing
4/5 The Marina, Harbour Road, Lydney, Gloucestershire, GL15 5ET

The contents of this book are for information only and are not intended as a substitute for appropriate medical attention. The author and publishers admit no liability for any consequences arising from following any advice contained within this book. If you have any concerns about your health or medication, always consult your doctor.

ISBN 1 904439 04 7

Printed and bound in Hong Kong through Printworks International Ltd.